# *Pegan Diet Dessert Recipe Book*

A Complete, Step-by-Step Cookbook

for Your Homemade Pegan Desserts

**Kimberly Solis**

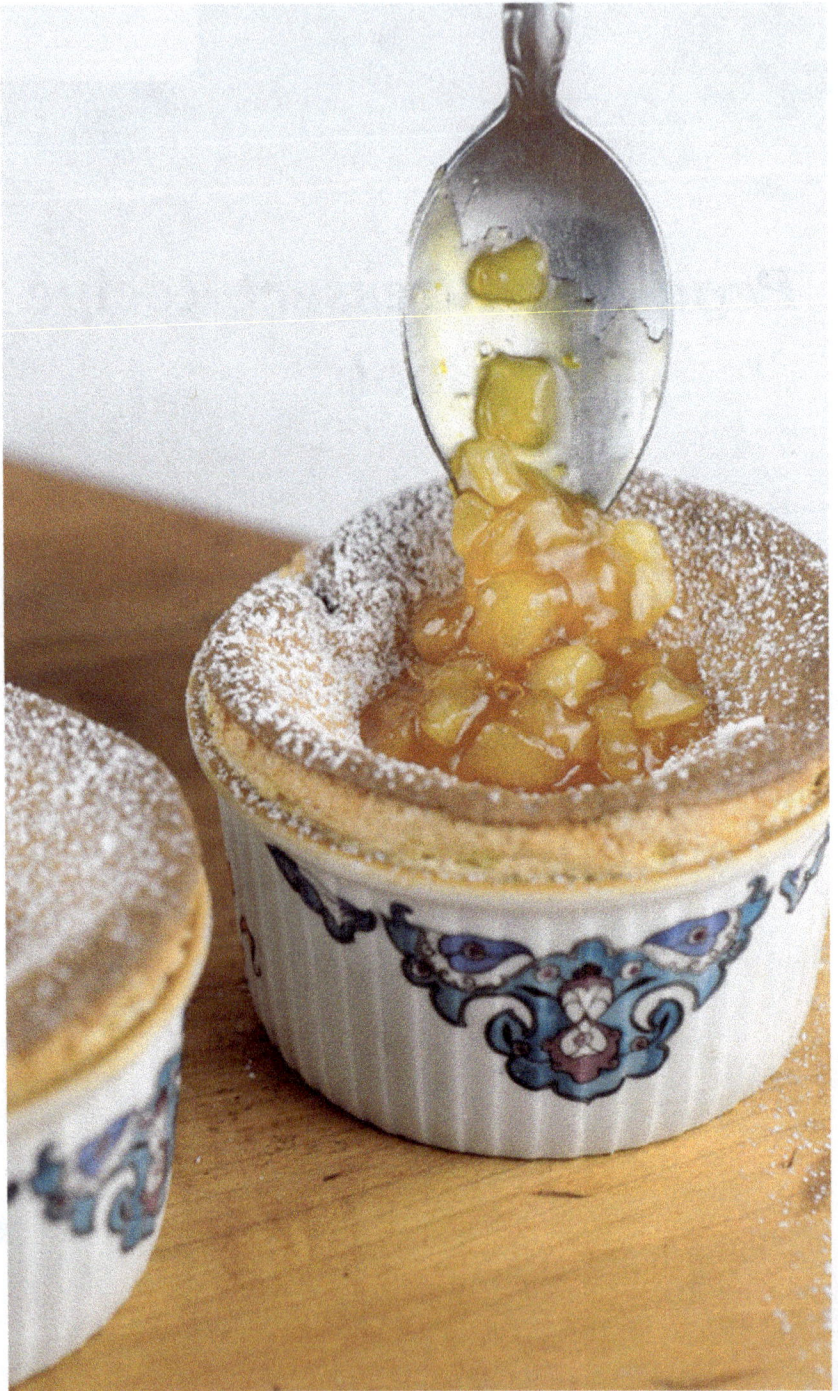

# Table of Contents

# Raspberry Brule

**Preparation Time:** 15 minutes

**Cooking Time:** 1 minute

**Servings:** 4

**Ingredients:**

- Light sour cream – ½ cup

- Plain cream cheese – ½ cup

- Brown sugar – ¼ cup, divided

- Ground cinnamon – ¼ tsp.

- Fresh raspberries – 1 cup

**Directions:**

1. Preheat the oven to broil.

2. In a bowl, beat together the cream cheese, sour cream, 2 tbsp. brown sugar and cinnamon for 4 minutes or until the mixture are very smooth and fluffy.

3. Evenly divide the raspberries among 4 (4-ounce) ramekins.

4. Spoon the cream cheese mixture over the berries and smooth the tops.

5. Sprinkle ½ tbsp. brown sugar evenly over each ramekin.

6. Place the ramekins on a baking sheet and broil 4 inches from the heating element until the sugar is caramelized and golden brown.

7. Cool and serve.

**Nutrition:**

Calories: 188;

Fat: 13g;

Carb: 16g;

Phosphorus: 60mg;

Potassium: 158mg;

Sodium: 132mg;

# Tart Apple Granita

**Preparation Time:** 15 minutes, plus 4 hours freezing time

**Cooking Time:** 0

**Servings:** 4

**Ingredients:**

- ½ cup granulated sugar

- ½ cup of water

- 2 cups unsweetened apple juice

- ¼ cup freshly squeezed lemon juice

**Directions:**

1. In a small saucepan over medium-high heat, heat the sugar and water.

2. Bring the mixture to a boil and then reduce the heat to low. Let it simmer for about 15 minutes or until the liquid has reduced by half.

3. Remove the pan from the heat and pour the liquid into a large shallow metal pan.

4. Let the liquid cool for about 30 minutes, and then stir in the apple juice and lemon juice.

5. Place the pan in the freezer.

6. After 1 hour, run a fork through the liquid to break up any ice crystals that have formed. Scrape down the sides as well.

7. Place the pan back in the freezer and repeat the stirring and scraping every 20 minutes, creating slush.

8. Serve when the mixture is completely frozen and looks like crushed ice, after about 3 hours.

**Nutrition:**

Calories: 157;

Fat: 0g;

Carbohydrates: 0g;

Phosphorus: 10mg;

Potassium: 141mg;

Sodium: 5mg;

Protein: 0g

# Lemon-Lime Sherbet

**Preparation Time:** 5 minutes, plus 3 hours chilling time

**Cooking Time:** 15 minutes

**Servings:** 2

**Ingredients:**

- 2 cups of water

- 1 cup granulated sugar

- 3 tablespoons lemon zest, divided

- ½ cup freshly squeezed lemon juice

- Zest of 1 lime

- Juice of 1 lime

- ½ cup heavy (whipping) cream

**Directions:**

1. Place a large saucepan over medium-high heat and add the water, sugar, and two tablespoons of the lemon zest.

2. Bring the mixture to a boil and then reduce the heat and simmer for 15 minutes.

3. Transfer the mixture to a large bowl and add the remaining 1 tablespoon lemon zest, the lemon juice, lime zest, and lime juice.

4. Chill the mixture in the fridge until completely cold, about 3 hours.

5. Whisk in the heavy cream and transfer the mixture to an ice cream maker.

6. Freeze according to the manufacturer's instructions.

**Nutrition:**

Calories: 151;

Fat: 6g;

Carbohydrates: 26g;

Phosphorus: 10mg;

Potassium: 27mg;

Sodium: 6mg;

Protein: 0g

# *Pavlova with Peaches*

**Preparation Time:** 30 minutes

**Cooking Time:** 1 hour, plus cooling time

**Servings: 3**

**Ingredients:**

- 4 large egg whites, at room temperature

- ½ teaspoon cream of tartar

- 1 cup superfine sugar

- ½ teaspoon pure vanilla extract

- 2 cups drained canned peaches in juice

**Directions:**

1. Preheat the oven to 225°F.

2. Line a baking sheet with parchment paper; set aside.

3. In a large bowl, beat the egg whites for about 1 minute or until soft peaks form.

4. Beat in the cream of tartar.

5. Add the sugar, one tablespoon at a time, until the egg whites are very stiff and glossy. Do not overbeat.

6. Beat in the vanilla.

7. Evenly spoon the meringue onto the baking sheet so that you have eight rounds.

8. Use the back of the spoon to create an indentation in the middle of each round.

9. Bake the meringues for about 1 hour or until a light brown crust form.

10. Turn off the oven and let the meringues stand, still in the oven, overnight.

11. Remove the meringues from the sheet and place them on serving plates.

12. Spoon the peaches, dividing evenly into the centers of the meringues and serve.

13. Store any unused meringues in a sealed container at room temperature for up to 1 week.

**Nutrition:**

Calories: 132;

Fat: 0g;

Carbohydrates: 32g;

Phosphorus: 7mg;

Potassium: 95mg;

Sodium: 30mg;

Protein: 2g

# *Tropical Vanilla*

**Preparation Time:** 15 minutes, plus freezing time

**Cooking Time:** 0 minutes

**Servings:** 2

**Ingredients:**

- 1 cup pineapple

- 1 cup of frozen strawberries

- 6 tablespoons water

- 2 tablespoons granulated sugar

- 1 tablespoon vanilla extract

**Directions:**

1. In a large saucepan, mix together the peaches, pineapple, strawberries, water, and sugar over medium-high heat and bring to a boil.

2. Reduce the heat to low and simmer the mixture, occasionally stirring, for 15 minutes.

3. Remove from the heat and let the mixture cool completely, for about 1 hour.

4. Stir in the vanilla and transfer the fruit mixture to a food processor or blender.

5. Purée until smooth, and pour the purée into a 9-by-13-inch glass baking dish.

6. Cover and place the dish in the freezer overnight.

7. When the fruit mixture is completely frozen, use a fork to scrape the sorbet until you have flaked flavored ice.

8. Scoop the ice flakes into four serving dishes.

**Nutrition:**

Calories: 92;

Fat: 0g;

Carbohydrates: 22g;

Phosphorus: 17mg;

Potassium: 145mg;

Sodium: 4mg;

Protein: 1g

# Rhubarb Crumble

**Preparation Time:** 15 minutes

**Cooking Time:** 30 minutes

**Servings: 6**

**Ingredients:**

- Unsalted butter, for greasing the baking dish

- 1 cup all-purpose flour

- ½ cup brown sugar

- ½ teaspoon ground cinnamon

- ½ cup unsalted butter, at room temperature

- 1 cup chopped rhubarb

- 2 apples, peeled, cored, and sliced thin

- 2 tablespoons granulated sugar

- 2 tablespoons water

**Directions:**

1. Preheat the oven to 325°F.

2. Lightly grease an 8-by-8-inch baking dish with butter; set aside.

3. In a small bowl, stir together the flour, sugar, and cinnamon until well combined.

4. Add the butter and rub the mixture between your fingers until it resembles coarse crumbs.

5. In a medium saucepan, mix together the rhubarb, apple, sugar, and water over medium heat and cook for about 20 minutes or until the rhubarb is soft.

6. Spoon the fruit mixture into the baking dish and evenly top with the crumble.

7. Bake the crumble for 20 to 30 minutes or until golden brown.

8. Serve hot.

**Nutrition:**

Calories: 450;

Fat: 23g;

Carbohydrates: 60g;

Phosphorus: 51mg;

Potassium: 181mg;

Sodium: 10mg;

Protein: 4g

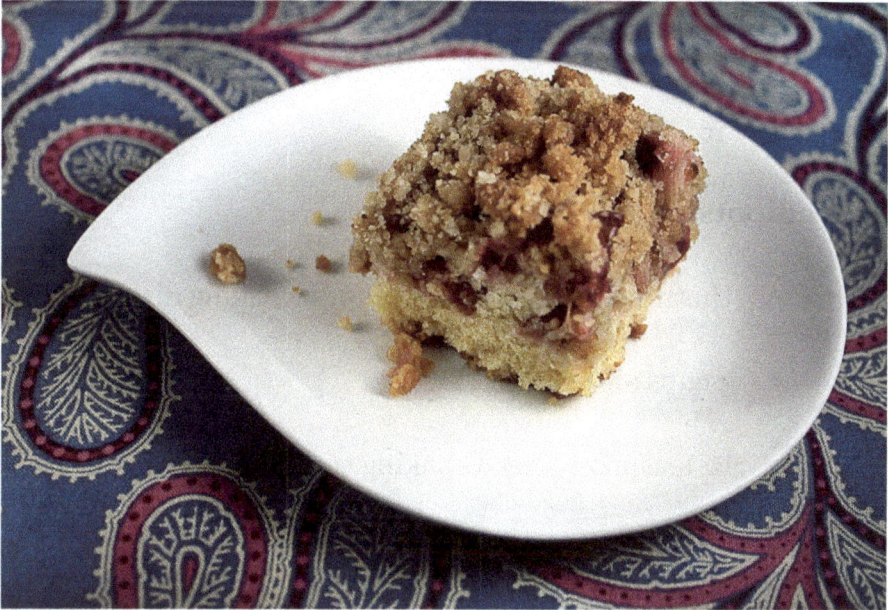

# Gingerbread Loaf

**Preparation Time:** 20 minutes

**Cooking Time:** 1 hour

**Servings:** 16

**Ingredients:**

- Unsalted butter, for greasing the baking dish

- 3 cups all-purpose flour

- ½ teaspoon Ener-G baking soda substitute

- 2 teaspoons ground cinnamon

- 1 teaspoon ground allspice

- ¾ cup granulated sugar

- 1¼ cups plain rice milk

- 1 large egg

- ¼ cup olive oil

- 2 tablespoons molasses

- 2 teaspoons grated fresh ginger

- Powdered sugar, for dusting

**Directions:**

1. Preheat the oven to 350°F.

2. Lightly grease a 9-by-13-inch baking dish with butter; set aside.

3. In a large bowl, sift together the flour, baking soda substitute, cinnamon, and allspice.

4. Stir the sugar into the flour mixture.

5. In medium bowl, whisk together the milk, egg, olive oil, molasses, and ginger until well blended.

6. Make a well in the center of the flour mixture and pour in the wet **Ingredients**.

7. Mix until just combined, taking care not to overmix.

8. Pour the batter into the baking dish and bake for about 1 hour or until a wooden pick inserted in the middle comes out clean.

9. Serve warm with a dusting of powdered sugar.

**Nutrition:**

Calories: 232;

Fat: 5g;

Carbohydrates: 42g;

Phosphorus: 54mg;

Potassium: 104mg;

Sodium: 18mg;

Protein: 4g

# Elegant Lavender Cookies

**Preparation Time** : 10 minutes

**Cooking Time:** 15 minutes

**Servings:** Makes 24 cookies

**Ingredients:**

- 5 dried organic lavender flowers, the entire top of the flower

- ½ cup granulated sugar

- 1 cup unsalted butter, at room temperature

- 2 cups all-purpose flour

- 1 cup of rice flour

**Directions:**

1. Strip the tiny lavender flowers off the main stem carefully and place the flowers and granulated sugar into a food processor or blender. Pulse until the mixture is finely chopped.

2. In a medium bowl, cream together the butter and

lavender sugar until it is very fluffy.

3.  Mix the flours into the creamed mixture until the mixture resembles fine crumbs.

4.  Gather the dough together into a ball and then roll it into a long log.

5.  Wrap the cookie dough in plastic and refrigerate it for about 1 hour or until firm.

6.  Preheat the oven to 375°F.

7.  Slice the chilled dough into ¼-inch rounds and refrigerate it for 1 hour or until firm.

8.  Bake the cookies for 15 to 18 minutes or until they are a very pale, golden brown.

9.  Let the cookies cool.

10. Store the cookies at room temperature in a sealed container for up to 1 week.

## Nutrition:

Calories: 153;

Fat: 9g;

Carbohydrates: 17g;

Phosphorus: 18mg;

Potassium: 17mg;

Sodium: 0mg;

Protein: 1g

# Carob Angel Food Cake

**Preparation Time:** 30 minutes

**Cooking Time:** 30 minutes

**Servings:** 16

**Ingredients:**

- ¾ cup all-purpose flour

- ¼ cup carob flour

- 1½ cups sugar, divided

- 12 large egg whites, at room temperature

- 1½ teaspoons cream of tartar

- 2 teaspoons vanilla

**Directions:**

1. Preheat the oven to 375°F.

2. In a medium bowl, sift together the all-purpose flour, carob flour, and ¾ cup of the sugar; set aside.

3. Beat the egg whites and cream of tartar with a hand mixer for about 5 minutes or until soft peaks form.

4.  Add the remaining ¾ cup sugar by the tablespoon to the egg whites until all the sugar is used up and stiff peaks form.

5.  Fold in the flour mixture and vanilla.

6.  Spoon the batter into an angel food cake pan.

7.  Run a knife through the batter to remove any air pockets.

8.  Bake the cake for about 30 minutes or until the top springs back when pressed lightly.

9.  Invert the pan onto a wire rack to cool.

10. Run a knife around the rim of the cake pan and remove the cake from the pan.

**Nutrition:**

Calories: 113;

Fat: 0g;

Carbohydrates: 25g;

Phosphorus: 11mg;

Potassium: 108mg;

Sodium: 42mg;

Protein: 3g

# Old-Fashioned Apple Kuchen

**Preparation Time** : 25 minutes

**Cook time:** 1 hour

**Servings:** 16

**Ingredients:**

- Unsalted butter, for greasing the baking dish

- 1 cup unsalted butter, at room temperature

- 2 cups granulated sugar

- 2 eggs, beaten

- 2 teaspoons pure vanilla extract

- 2 cups all-purpose flour

- 1 teaspoon Ener-G baking soda substitute

- 2 teaspoons ground cinnamon

- ½ teaspoon ground nutmeg

- Pinch ground allspice

- 2 large apples, peeled, cored, and diced (about 3 cups)

**Directions:**

1. Preheat the oven to 350°F.

2. Grease a 9-by-13-inch glass baking dish; set aside.

3. Cream together the butter and sugar with a hand mixer until light and fluffy, for about 3 minutes.

4. Add the eggs and vanilla and beat until combined, scraping down the sides of the bowl, about 1 minute.

5. In a small bowl, stir together the flour, baking soda substitute, cinnamon, nutmeg, and allspice.

6. Add the dry **Ingredients** to the wet **Ingredients** and stir to combine.

7. Stir in the apple and spoon the batter into the baking dish.

8. Bake for about 1 hour or until the cake is golden.

9. Cool the cake on a wire rack.

10. Serve warm or chilled.

**Nutrition:**

Calories: 368;

Fat: 16g;

Carbohydrates: 53g;

Phosphorus: 46mg;

Potassium: 68mg;

Sodium: 15mg;

Protein: 3g

# Dark Chocolate and Cherry Trail Mix

**Preparation Time:** 5 minutes

**Cooking Time:** 5 minutes

**Servings:** Makes 3 cups (¼ cup per serving)

**Ingredients:**

- 1 cup unsalted almonds

- 2/3 cup dried cherries

- ½ cup walnuts

- ½ cup sweet cinnamon-roasted chickpeas

- ¼ cup dark chocolate chips

**Directions:**

1. Combine the almonds, cherries, walnuts, chickpeas, and chocolate chips in an airtight container.

2. Store at room temperature for up to 1 week or in the freezer for up to 3 months.

**Nutrition:**

Calories: 174;

Total Fat: 12g;

Saturated Fat: 2g;

Cholesterol: 0mg;

Sodium: 18mg;

Carbohydrates: 16g;

Fiber: 4g;

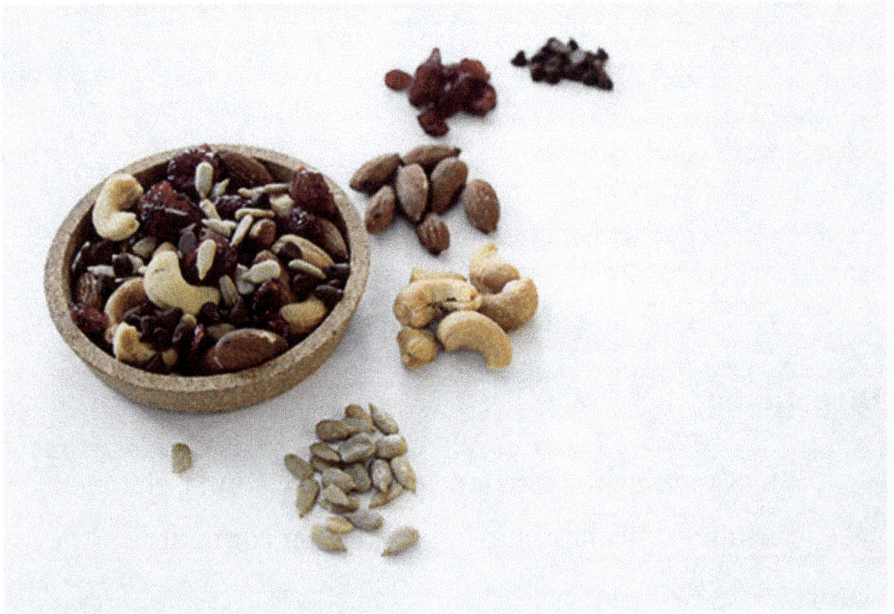

# *Coconut Balls*

**Preparation Time**: 10minutes

**Cooking Time**: 0minutes

**Servings**: 3

**Ingredients**:

- 1/3 cup coconut oil melted

- 1/3 cup coconut butter softened

- 2 oz. coconut, finely shredded, unsweetened

- 4 Tbsp. coconut palm sugar

- 1/2 cup shredded coconut

**Directions**:

1. Combine all **Ingredients** in a blender.

2. Blend until soft and well combined.

3. Do a small ball roll in shredded coconut.

4. Place on a sheet lined with parchment paper and refrigerate overnight.

5.  Keep coconut balls into sealed container in fridge up to one week.

**Nutrition**:

Calories 226.89

Calories from Fat 190.39 |

Total Fat 21.6g

Saturated Fat 19.84g

Cholesterol 0mg

Sodium 17.19mg

Potassium 45mg

Total Carbohydrates 9g

Fiber 1.16g

Sugar 5.7g

Protein 1g

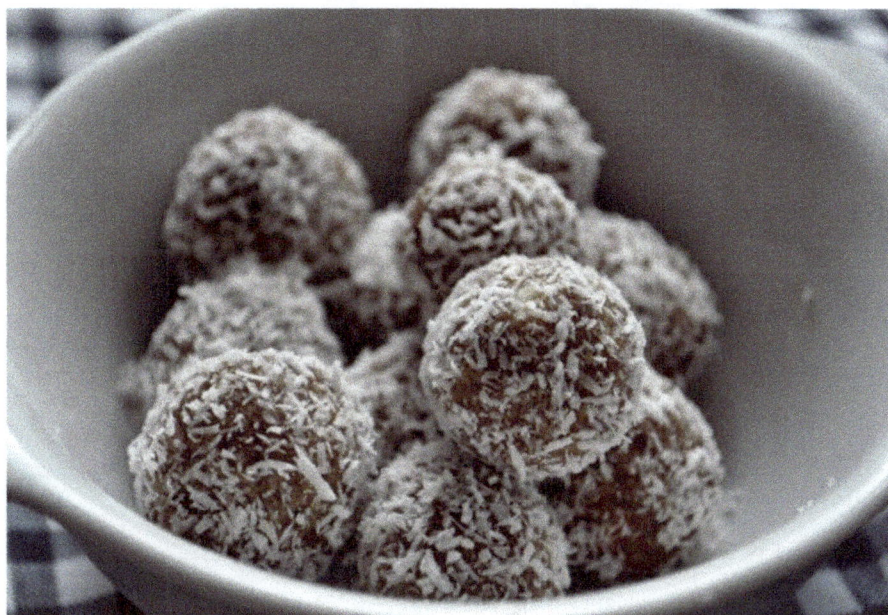

# Almond - Choco Cake

**Preparation Time**: 10minutes

**Cooking Time**: 45minutes

**Servings**: 5

**Ingredients***:*

- 1 1/2 cups of almond flour

- 1/3 cup almonds finely chopped

- 1/4 cup of cocoa powder unsweetened

- Pinch of salt

- 1/2 tsp. baking soda

- 2 Tbsp. almond milk

- 1/2 cup Coconut oil melted

- 2 tsp. pure vanilla extract

- 1/3 cup brown sugar (packed)

**Directions**:

1. Preheat oven to 350 F.

2. Set the pan, and grease with a little melted coconut oil; set aside.

3. Stir the almond flour, chopped almonds, cocoa powder, salt, and baking soda in a bowl.

4. In a separate bowl, stir the remaining **Ingredients**.

5. Merge the almond flour mixture with the almond milk mixture and stir well.

6. Place batter in a prepared cake pan.

7. Bake for 30 to 32 minutes…

8. Store the cake-slices a freezer, tightly wrapped in a double layer of plastic wrap and a layer of foil. It will keep on this way for up to a month.

**Nutrition**:

Calories 326.89

Calories from Fat 165.39 |

Total Fat 34.6g

Saturated Fat 29.84g

Cholesterol 0mg

Sodium 18.19mg

Potassium 45mg

Total Carbohydrates 9g

Fiber 1.16g

Sugar 5.7g

Protein 1g

# *Banana-Almond Cake*

**Preparation Time**: 10minutes

**Cooking Time**: 45minutes

**Servings**: 5

**Ingredients**

- 4 ripe bananas in chunks

- 3 Tbsps. honey or maple syrup

- 1 tsp. pure vanilla extract

- 1/2 cup almond milk

- 3/4 cup of self-rising flour

- 1 tsp. cinnamon

- 1 tsp. baking powder

- 1 pinch of salt

- 1/3 cup of almonds finely chopped

- Almond slices for decoration

**Directions**:

1.  Preheat the oven to 400 F (air mode).

2.  Oil a cake mold; set aside.

3.  Add bananas into a bowl and mash with the fork.

4.  Add honey, vanilla, almond, and stir well.

5.  In a separate bowl, stir flour, cinnamon, baking powder, salt, the almonds broken, and mix with a spoon.

6.  Transfer the mixture to prepared cake mold and sprinkle with sliced almonds.

7.  Bake for 40-45 minutes.

8.  Remove from the oven, and allow the cake to cool completely.

9.  Cut cake into slices, place in tin foil, or an airtight container, and keep refrigerated up to one week.

**Nutrition**:

Calories 326.89

Calories from Fat 145.39 |

Total Fat 24.6g

Saturated Fat 12.84g

Cholesterol 0mg

Sodium 20.19mg

Potassium 32

Total Carbohydrates 9g

Fiber 1.16g

Sugar 5.7g

Protein 1g

# *Banana-Coconut Ice Cream*

**Preparation Time**: 15minutes

**Cooking Time**: 0minutes

**Servings**: 5

**Ingredients**

- 1 cup coconut cream

- 1/2 cup Inverted sugar

- 2 large frozen bananas (chunks)

- 3 Tbsp. honey extracted

- 1/4 tsp. cinnamon powder

**Directions**:

1. Do the coconut cream with the inverted sugar in a bowl.

2. In a separate bowl, beat the banana with honey and cinnamon.

3. Incorporate the coconut whipped cream and banana mixture; stir well.

4. Cover the bowl and let cool in the refrigerator over the night.

5. Stir the mixture 3 to 4 times to avoid crystallization.

6. Keep frozen 1 to 2 months.

**Nutrition**:

Calories 126.89

Calories from Fat 245.39 |

Total Fat 34.6g

Saturated Fat 12.84g

Cholesterol 0mg

Sodium 20.19mg

Potassium 32

Total Carbohydrates 9g

Fiber 1.16g

Sugar 5.7g

Protein 1g

# Coconut Butter Clouds Cookies

**Preparation Time**: 15minutes

**Cooking Time**: 25minutes

**Servings**: 5

**Ingredients**

- 1/2 cup coconut butter softened

- 1/2 cup peanut butter softened

- 1/2 cup of granulated sugar

- 1/2 cup of brown sugar

- 2 Tbsp. chia seeds soaked in 4 tablespoons water

- 1/2 tsp. pure vanilla extract

- 1/2 tsp. baking soda

- 1/4 tsp. salt

- 1 cup of all-purpose flour

**Directions**:

1. Preheat oven to 360 F.

2. Add coconut butter, peanut butter, and both sugars in a mixing bowl.

3. Beat with a mixer until soft and sugar combined well.

4. Add soaked chia seeds and vanilla extract; beat.

5. Add baking soda, salt, and flour; beat until all **Ingredients** are combined well.

6. With your hands, shape dough into cookies.

7. Arrange your cookies onto a baking sheet, and bake for about 10 minutes.

8. Remove cookies from the oven and allow cooling completely.

9. Sprinkle with icing sugar and enjoy your cookies.

10. Place cookies in an airtight container and keep refrigerated up to 10 days.

## Nutrition:

Calories 226.89

Calories from Fat 255.39 |

Total Fat 34.6g

Saturated Fat 12.84g

Cholesterol 0mg

Sodium 10.19mg

Potassium 22

Total Carbohydrates 10g

Fiber 1.16g

Sugar 7.7g

Protein 5g

# *Choco Mint Hazelnut Bars*

**Preparation Time**: 15minutes

**Cooking Time**: 35minutes

**Servings**: 4

**Ingredients**

- 1/2 cup coconut oil, melted

- 4 Tbsp. cocoa powder

- 1/4 cup almond butter

- 3/4 cup brown sugar - (packed)

- 1 tsp. vanilla extract

- 1 tsp. pure peppermint extract

- Pinch of salt

- 1 cup shredded coconut

- 1 cup hazelnuts sliced

**Directions**:

1. Slice the hazelnuts in a food processor

2. Boil the and place it on low heat.

3. Put the coconut oil, cacao powder, almond butter, brown sugar, vanilla, peppermint extract, and salt in the top of a double boiler over hot (not boiling) water and constantly stir for 10 minutes.

4. Add hazelnuts and shredded coconut to the melted mixture and stir together.

5. Pour the mixture in a dish lined with parchment and freeze for several hours.

6. Remove from the freezer and cut into bars.

7. Store in airtight container or freezer bag in a freezer.

8. Let the bars at room temperature for 10 to 15 minutes before eating.

**Nutrition**:

Calories 126.89

Calories from Fat 155.39 |

Total Fat 34.6g

Saturated Fat 18.84g

Cholesterol 0mg

Sodium 15.19mg

Potassium 32

Total Carbohydrates 10g

Fiber 1.16g

Sugar 7.7g

Protein 5g

# Coco-Cinnamon Balls

**Preparation Time**: 15minutes

**Cooking Time**: 35minutes

**Servings**: 4

**Ingredients**

- 1 cup coconut butter softened

- 1 cup coconut milk canned

- 1 tsp. pure vanilla extract

- 3/4 tsp. cinnamon

- 1/2 tsp. nutmeg

- 2 Tbsp. coconut palm sugar (or granulated sugar)

- 1 cup coconut shreds

**Directions**:

1. Combine all **Ingredients** (except the coconut shreds) in a heated bath - bain-marie.

2. Cook and stir until all **Ingredients** are soft and well combined.

3. Remove bowl from heat, place into a bowl, and refrigerate until the mixture firmed up.

4. Form cold coconut mixture into balls, and roll each ball in the shredded coconut.

5. Store into a sealed container, and keep refrigerated up to one week.

**Nutrition**:

Calories 136.89

Fat 235.39 |

Total Fat 24.6g

Saturated Fat 19.84g

Cholesterol 0mg

Sodium 15.19mg

Potassium 32

Total Carbohydrates 10g

Fiber 2.16g

Sugar 7.7g

Protein 5g

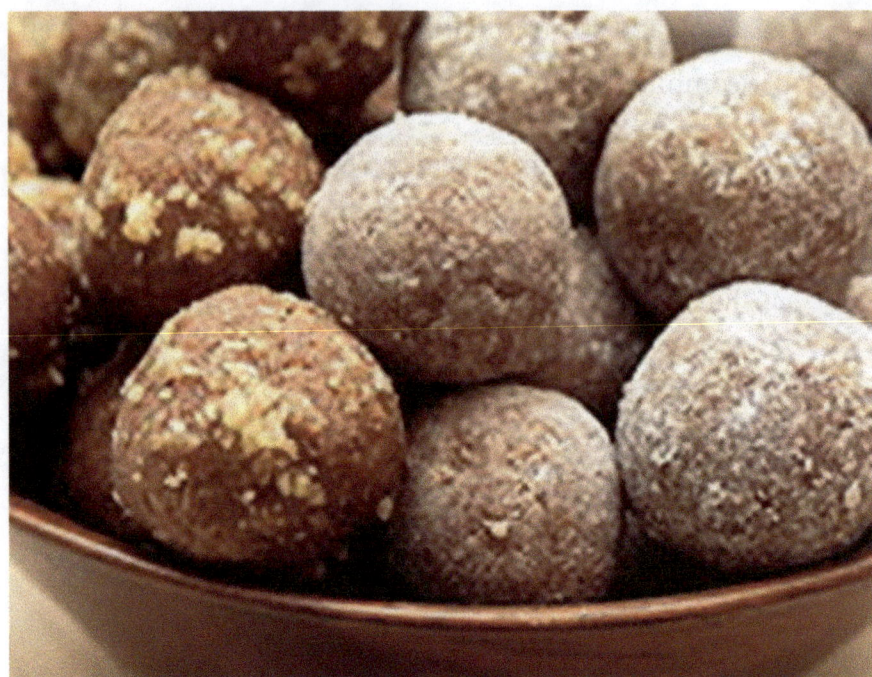

# Coconut Flax Pudding

**Preparation Time**: 15minutes

**Cooking Time**: 25minutes

**Servings**: 4

**Ingredients**

- 1 Tbsp. coconut oil softened

- 1 Tbsp. coconut cream

- 2 cups coconut milk canned

- 3/4 cup ground flax seed

- 4 Tbsp. coconut palm sugar (or to taste)

**Directions**:

1. Press SAUTÉ button on your Pressure pot

2. Add coconut oil, coconut cream, coconut milk, and ground flaxseed.

3. Stir about 5 - 10 minutes.

4. Close lid into place and Start.

5. When the timer beeps, press "Cancel" and carefully flip the Quick Release valve to let the pressure out.

6. Add the palm sugar and stir well.

7. Taste and adjust sugar to taste.

8. Allow pudding to cool down completely.

9. Set the pudding in an airtight container and refrigerate for up to 2 weeks.

**Nutrition**:

Calories 126.89

Calories from Fat 124.39 |

Total Fat 14.6g

Saturated Fat 17.84g

Cholesterol 0mg

Sodium 18.19mg

Potassium 22

Total Carbohydrates 10g

Fiber 2.16g

Sugar 7.7g

Protein 5g

# Full-Flavored Vanilla Ice Cream

**Preparation Time**: 15minutes

**Cooking Time**: 0minutes

**Servings**: 4

**Ingredients**

- 1 1/2 cups canned coconut milk

- 1 cup coconut whipping cream

- 1 frozen banana cut into chunks

- 1 cup vanilla sugar

- 3 Tbsp. apple sauce

- 2 tsp. pure vanilla extract

- 1 tsp. Xanthan gum or agar-agar thickening agent

**Directions**:

1. Merge all Ingredients; process until all Ingredients combined well.

2. Place the ice cream mixture in a freezer-safe container with a lid over.

3. Freeze for at least 4 hours.

4. Remove frozen mixture to a bowl and beat with a mixer to break up the ice crystals.

5. Repeat this process 3 to 4 times.

6. Let the ice cream at room temperature for 15 minutes before serving.

**Nutrition**:

Calories 126.89

Calories from Fat 134.39 |

Total Fat 15.6g

Saturated Fat 19.84g

Cholesterol 0mg

Sodium 28.19mg

Potassium 22

Total Carbohydrates 10g

Fiber 2.16g

Sugar 7.7g

Protein 5g

# Irresistible Peanut Cookies

**Preparation Time**: 20minutes

**Cooking Time**: 0minutes

**Servings**: 6

**Ingredients**

- 4 Tbsp. all-purpose flour

- 1 tsp. baking soda

- Pinch of salt

- 1/3 cup granulated sugar

- 1/3 cup peanut butter softened

- 3 Tbsp. applesauce

- 1/2 tsp. pure vanilla extract

**Directions**:

1. Preheat oven to 350 F.

2. Combine the flour, baking soda, salt, and sugar in a mixing bowl; stir.

3. Merge all remaining **Ingredients**

4. Roll dough into cookie balls/patties.

5. Arrange your cookies onto greased (with oil or cooking spray) baking sheet.

6. Let cool before removing from tray.

7. Take out cookies from the tray and let cool completely.

8. Place your peanut butter cookies in an airtight container, and keep refrigerated up to 10 days.

**Nutrition**:

Calories 116.89

Calories from Fat 114.39 |

Total Fat 18.6g

Saturated Fat 20.84g

Cholesterol 0mg

Sodium 12.19mg

Potassium 22

Total Carbohydrates 10g

Fiber 2.16g

Sugar 7.7g

Protein 5g

# *Murky Almond Cookies*

**Preparation Time**: 10minutes

**Cooking Time**: 15minutes

**Servings**: 6

**Ingredients**

- 4 Tbsp. cocoa powder

- 2 cups almond flour

- 1/4 tsp. salt

- 1/2 tsp. baking soda

- 5 Tbsp. coconut oil melted

- 2 Tbsp. almond milk

- 1 1/2 tsp. almond extract

- 1 tsp. vanilla extract

- 4 Tbsp. corn syrup or honey

**Directions**:

1. Preheat oven to 340 F degrees.

2. Grease a large baking sheet; set aside.

3. Merge the cocoa powder, almond flour, salt, and baking soda.

4. Merge the melted coconut oil, almond milk; almond and vanilla extract, and corn syrup or honey.

5. Merge the almond flour mixture with the almond milk mixture and stir well.

6. Roll tablespoons of the dough into balls, and arrange onto a prepared baking sheet.

7. Bake for 12 to 15 minutes.

8. Remove from the oven and transfer onto a plate lined with a paper towel.

9. Allow cookies to cool down completely and store in an airtight container at room temperature for about four days.

**Nutrition**:

Calories 16.89

Calories from Fat 19.39 |

Total Fat 18.6g

Saturated Fat 20.84g

Cholesterol 0mg

Sodium 12.19mg

Potassium 22

Total Carbohydrates 10g

Fiber 2.16g

Sugar 7.7g

Protein 5g

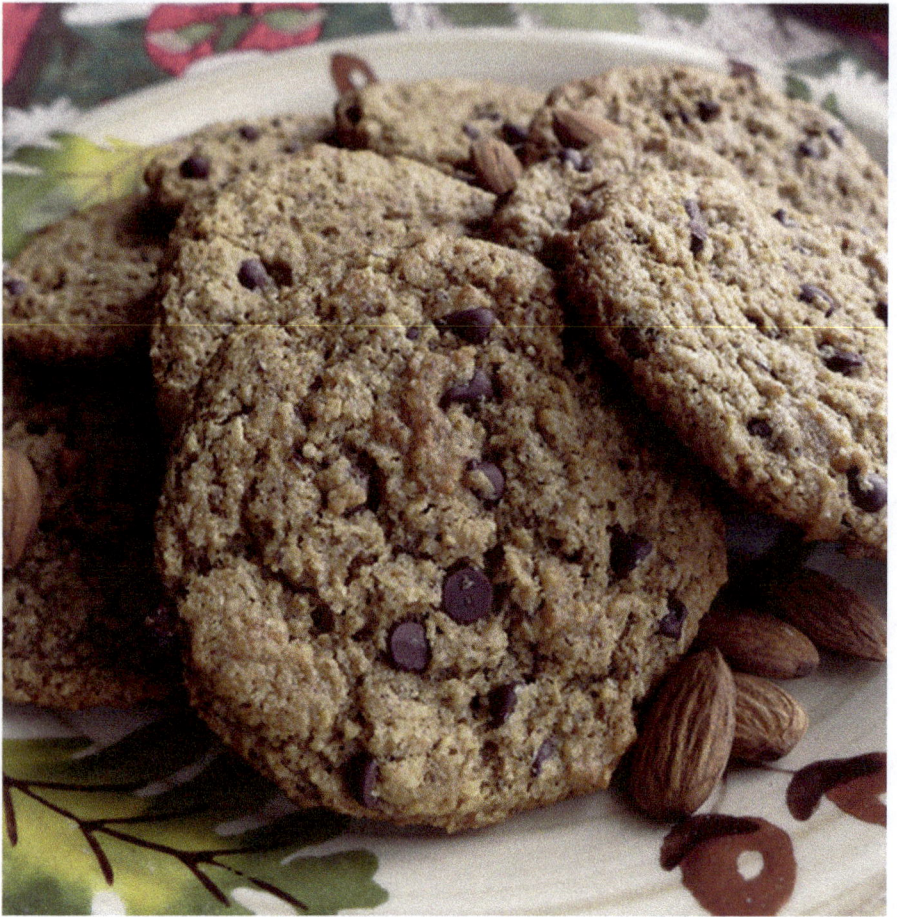

# Orange Semolina Halva

**Preparation Time**: 10minutes

**Cooking Time**: 25minutes

**Servings**: 6

**Ingredients**

- 6 cups fresh orange juice

- Zest from 3 oranges

- 3 cups brown sugar

- 1 1/4 cup semolina flour

- 1 Tbsp. almond butter (plain, unsalted)

- 4 Tbsp. ground almond

- 1/4 tsp. cinnamon

**Directions**:

1. Heat the orange juice, orange zest with brown sugar in a pot.

2. Let the sugar dissolved.

3.  Add the semolina flour and cook over low heat for 15 minutes; stir occasionally.

4.  Add almond butter, ground almonds, and cinnamon, and stir well.

5.  Cook, frequently stirring, for further 5 minutes.

6.  Transfer the halva mixture into a mold, let it cool and refrigerate for at least 4 hours.

7.  Keep refrigerated in a sealed container for one week.

**Nutrition**:

Calories 16.89

Calories from Fat 19.39 |

Total Fat 18.6g

Saturated Fat 20.84g

Cholesterol 0mg

Sodium 12.19mg

Potassium 22

Total Carbohydrates 10g

Fiber 2.16g

Sugar 7.7g

Protein 5g

# Seasoned Cinnamon Mango Popsicles

**Preparation Time**: 15minutes

**Cooking Time**: 0minutes

**Servings**: 6

**Ingredients**

- 1 1/2 cups of mango pulp

- 1 mango cut in cubes

- 1 cup brown sugar (packed)

- 2 Tbsp. lemon juice freshly squeezed

- 1 tsp. cinnamon

- 1 pinch of salt

**Directions**:

1. Add all **Ingredients** into your blender.

2. Blend until brown sugar dissolved.

3. Pour the mango mixture evenly in Popsicle molds or cups.

4. Insert sticks into each mold.

5. Place molds in a freezer, and freeze for at least 5 to6 hours.

6. Before serving, un-mold easy your popsicles placing molds under lukewarm water.

**Nutrition**:

Calories 16.89

Calories from Fat 19.39 |

Total Fat 18.6g

Saturated Fat 20.84g

Cholesterol 0mg

Sodium 12.19mg

Potassium 22

Total Carbohydrates 10g

Fiber 2.16g

Sugar 7.7g

Protein 5g

# *Strawberry Molasses Ice Cream*

**Preparation Time**: 20minutes

**Cooking Time**: 0minutes

**Servings**: 9

**Ingredients**

- 1 lb. strawberries

- 3/4 cup coconut palm sugar

- 1 cup coconut cream

- 1 Tbsp. molasses

- 1 tsp. balsamic vinegar

- 1/2 tsp. agar-agar

- 1/2 tsp. pure strawberry extract

**Directions**:

1. Add strawberries, date sugar, and the balsamic vinegar in a blender; blend until completely combined.

2. Place the mixture in the refrigerator for one hour.

3. In a mixing bowl, beat the coconut cream with an electric mixer to make a thick mixture.

4. Add molasses, balsamic vinegar, agar-agar, and beat for further one minute or until combined well.

5. Add the strawberry mixture and beat again for 2 minutes.

6. Pour ice cream mix into an ice cream maker, turn on the machine, and churn according to manufacturer's **Directions**.

7. Keep frozen in a freezer-safe container (with plastic film and lid over).

**Nutrition**:

Calories 16.89

Calories from Fat 19.39 |

Total Fat 18.6g

Saturated Fat 20.84g

Cholesterol 0mg

Sodium 12.19mg

Potassium 22

Total Carbohydrates 10g

Fiber 2.16g

Sugar 7.7g

Protein 5g

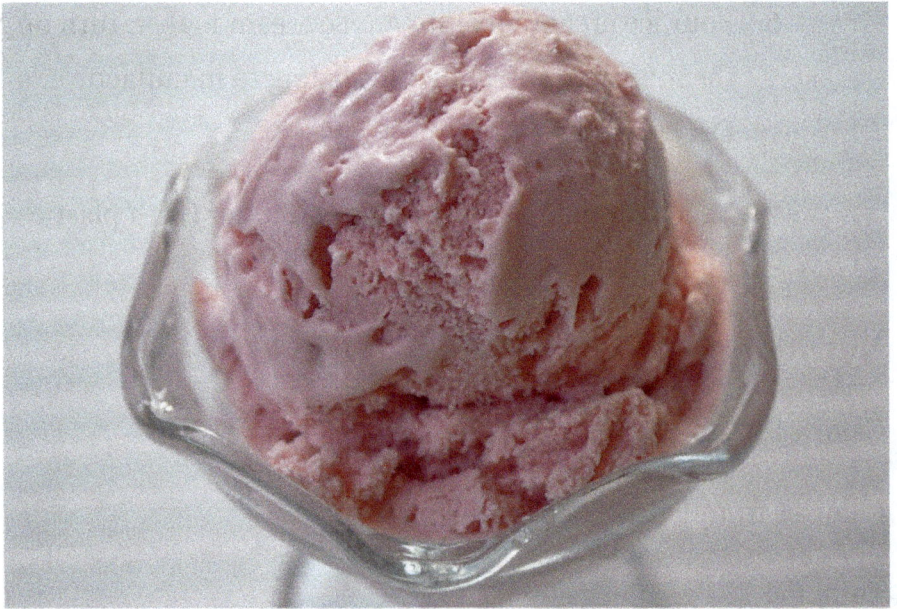

# *Strawberry-Mint Sorbet*

**Preparation Time**: 15minutes

**Cooking Time**: 0minutes

**Servings**: 6

**Ingredients**

- 1 cup of granulated sugar

- 1 cup of orange juice

- 1 lb. frozen strawberries

- 1 tsp. pure peppermint extract

**Directions**:

1. Add sugar and orange juice in a saucepan.

2. Stir over high heat and boil for 5 minutes or until sugar dissolves.

3. Remove from the heat and let it cool down.

4. Add strawberries into a blender, and blend until smooth.

5. Pour syrup into strawberries, add peppermint extract and stir until all **Ingredients** combined well.

6. Transfer mixture to a storage container, cover tightly, and freeze until ready to serve.

**Nutrition**:

Calories 16.89

Calories from Fat 1.39 |

Total Fat 12.6g

Saturated Fat 2.84g

Cholesterol 0mg

Sodium 1.19mg

Potassium 22

Total Carbohydrates 10g

Fiber 2.16g

Sugar 33g

Protein 5g

# Vegan Choco Spread

**Preparation Time**: 15minutes

**Cooking Time**: 0minutes

**Servings**: 5

**Ingredients**

- 1 cup hazelnuts soaked

- 4 Tbsp. dry cacao powder

- 4 Tbsp. Maple syrup

- 1 tsp. pure vanilla extract

- 1/4 tsp. kosher salt

- 4 Tbsp. almond milk

**Directions**:

1. Soak hazelnuts with water overnight.

2. Add soaked hazelnuts along with all remaining **Ingredients** in a food processor.

3. Process for about 10 minutes or until a cream gets the desired consistency.

4. Keep the spread in a sealed container refrigerated up to 2 weeks.

**Nutrition**:

Calories 16.89

Calories from Fat 4.39 |

Total Fat 6.6g

Saturated Fat 3.84g

Cholesterol 0mg

Sodium 5.19mg

Potassium 22

Total Carbohydrates 10g

Fiber 2.16g

Sugar 43g

Protein 5g

# Vegan Exotic Chocolate Mousse

**Preparation Time**: 10minutes

**Cooking Time**: 0minutes

**Servings**: 4

**Ingredients**:

- 2 frozen bananas chunks

- 2 avocados

- 1/3 cup of dates

- 4 Tbsp. cocoa powder

- 1/2 cup of fresh orange juice

- Zest, from 1 orange

**Directions**:

1. Add bananas, avocado, and dates in a food processor.

2. Process for about 2 to 3 minutes until combined well.

3. Add cocoa powder, orange juice, and orange zest; process for further one minute.

4. Place cream in a glass jar or container and keep refrigerated up to one week.

**Nutrition**:

Calories 16.89

Calories from Fat 4.39 |

Total Fat 5.6g

Saturated Fat 2.84g

Cholesterol 0mg

Sodium 7.19mg

Potassium 32

Total Carbohydrates 10g

Fiber 2.16g

Sugar 43g

Protein 5g

# *Vegan Lemon Pudding*

**Preparation Time**: 20minutes

**Cooking Time**: 0minutes

**Servings**: 6

**Ingredients**

- 2 cups almond milk

- 3 Tbsp. of corn flour

- 2 Tbsp. of all-purpose flour

- 1 cup of sugar granulated

- 1/4 cup almond butter (plain, unsalted)

- 1 tsp. lemon zest

- 1/3 cup fresh lemon juice

**Directions**:

1. Add the almond milk with corn flour, flour, and sugar in a saucepan.

2. Cook, frequently stirring, until sugar dissolved, and all **Ingredients** combine well (for about 5 to 7 minutes over medium heat).

3. Add the almond butter, lemon zest, and lemon juice.

4. Cook, frequently stirring, for further 5 to 6 minutes.

5. Remove the lemon pudding from the heat and allow it to cool completely.

6. Pour into the sealed container and keep refrigerated up to one week.

**Nutrition**:

Calories 16.89

Calories from Fat 7.39 |

Total Fat 3.6g

Saturated Fat 1.84g

Cholesterol 0mg

Sodium 7.19mg

Potassium432

Total Carbohydrates 20g

Fiber 1.16g

Sugar 24g

Protein 5g

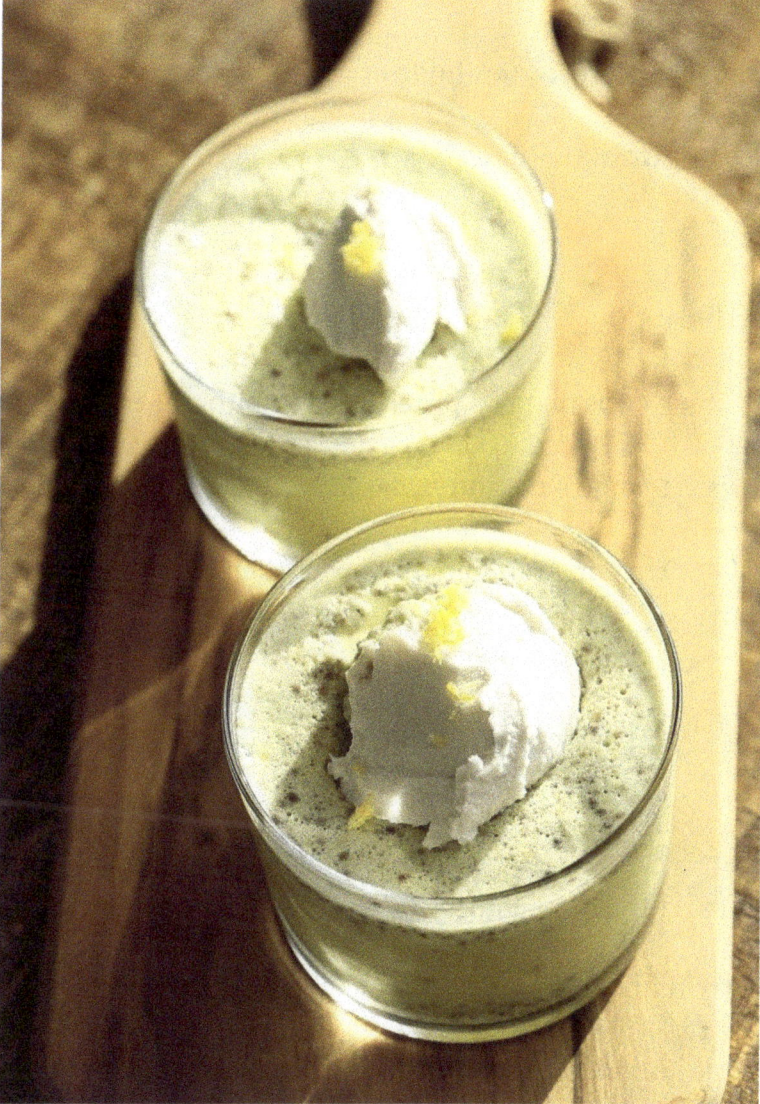

# *Vitamin Blast Tropical Sherbet*

**Preparation Time**: 15minutes

**Cooking Time**: 0minutes

**Servings**: 8

**Ingredients**

- 4 cups mangos pitted and cut into 1/2-inch dice

- 1 papaya cut into 1/2-inch dice

- 1/4 cup granulated sugar or honey (optional)

- 1 cup pineapple juice canned

- 1/4 cup coconut milk

- 2 Tbsp. coconut cream

- 1 fresh lime juice

**Directions**:

1. Add all **Ingredients** into your food processor; process until all **Ingredients** smooth and combine well.

2. Put the mixture to a bowl, and cover

3. Remove the sherbet mixture from the fridge, stir well, and pour in a freezer-safe container (with plastic film and lid over).

4. Keep frozen.

5. Let the sherbet at room temperature for 15 minutes before serving.

**Nutrition**:

Calories 16.89

Calories from Fat 9.39 |

Total Fat 2.6g

Saturated Fat 3.84g

Cholesterol 0mg

Sodium 7.15mg

Potassium132

Total Carbohydrates 15g

Fiber 1.16g

Sugar 24g

Protein 5g

# *Walnut Vanilla Popsicles*

**Preparation Time**: 15minutes

**Cooking Time**: 0minutes

**Servings**: 7

**Ingredients**

- 1 1/2 cup finely sliced walnuts

- 4 cups of almond milk

- 4 Tbsp. brown sugar (packed)

- 1 scoop protein powder (pea or soy)

- 2 tsp. pure vanilla extract

**Directions**:

1. Add all **Ingredients** in your high-speed blender and blend until smooth and combined well.

2. Pour the mixture in Popsicle molds and insert the wooden stick into the middle of each mold.

3. Freeze until your ice popsicles are completely frozen.

4. Serve and enjoy!

**Nutrition**:

Calories 16.89

Calories from Fat 9.39 |

Total Fat 2.6g

Saturated Fat 3.84g

Cholesterol 0mg

Sodium 7.15mg

Potassium122

Total Carbohydrates 15g

Fiber 1.16g

Sugar 34g

Protein 5g

# Sun Dried Tomato Pesto Mug Cake

**Servings** 1 Sun Dried Tomato Pesto Mug Cake

## Ingredients

- Base
- 1 large egg
- 2 tablespoons butter
- 2 tablespoons almond flour
- ½ teaspoon baking powder
- 5 teaspoons sun dried tomato pesto 1 tablespoon almond flour
- Pinch salt

## Instructions

1. Get your mug ready! Add 1 Large Egg, 3 Tbsp. Honeyville Almond Flour, 2 Tbsp. of Room Temperature Butter, 5 tsp. Sun Dried Tomato Pesto, 1/2 tsp. Baking Powder and a pinch of salt.
2. Mix everything together well.
3. Microwave this for 75 seconds on high (power level 10).

4. Then, lightly slam your mug against a plate so that it comes out. Top with extra cheese sun dried tomato and a small wedge of fresh tomato!

## Nutrition Info

429 Calories 40.45g Fats 5.32g Net Carbs 12.34g Protein

# *Peanut Butter Granola Balls*

**Prep Time**: 10 mins

**Total Time**: 20 mins

**Servings**: 12 granola balls

**Ingredients**

- Dry ingredients
- 1 cup Sliced almonds 1/4 cup Pumpkin seeds 1 tablespoon Chia seeds
- 2 tablespoon Flaxseed meal
- 1/4 cup Unsweetened desiccated Coconut 1/4 teaspoon Salt
- 1/4 cup Sugar-free Chocolate Chips or dark chocolate chips
- >85% cocoa or cocoa nibs Liquid ingredients
- 1/2 cup Natural Peanut butter smooth, unsalted
- 1/4 cup Sugar-free flavored maple syrup or liquid sweetener of choice


Chcoolate drizzle

1/4 cup Sugar-free Chocolate Chips 1/2 teaspoon Coconut oil

## Instructions

1. In a large mixing bowl add all the dry ingredients, stir to combine, set aside. Note: you can add the chocolate chips now and they will melt in the next step giving a chocolate peanut butter flavor to the ball or you can choose to add the chocolate chips after step 3 to keep the crunchy chocolate chips bites in the balls.

2. In a small bowl, add the liquid ingredients: peanut butter and sugar-free liquid sweetener, microwave 45 seconds. This step will soften the peanut butter making it easier to combine with the dry ingredients. Don't over-warm.

3. Pour the liquid ingredients onto the dry ingredients, combine using a spatula until it forms a sticky batter that you can easily shape into granola balls. If you didn't add the chocolate chips in step 1, stir in now.

4. Slightly grease your hands with coconut oil, grab some dough and roll the granola balls. I recommend a 'golf ball' size to make 12 granola balls in total with this batter.

5. Roll the prepared granola balls in extra sliced almonds if you like to add some crunch on the sides. Place the granola ball on a plate that you have covered with parchment paper - this prevents the ball from sticking to the plate.

6. Repeat the rolling process until you form 12 granola balls. Place the plate in the freezer for 10 minutes to firm up the

granola balls. Meanwhile melt the extra chocolate chips with coconut oil.

7. Remove the plate from the freezer, drizzle some melted chocolate on top of each granola ball. Place the plate in the freezer again for 5 minutes to set the chocolate drizzle.

8. Store up to 3 weeks in the fridge in an airtight container or up to 10 days in the pantry in a cookie jar.

**Nutrition Info**

Calories 145 Calories from Fat 107 Fat 11.9g Carbohydrates 7.5g Fiber 3.3g Sugar 1.5g Protein 5.3g

# *Chocolate Peanut Butter Chia Seed Pudding*

**Prep Time:** 10 mins

**Total Time**: 1 hr 10 mins

**Servings**: 6 pudding

- Ingredients
- 2/3 cup Chia seeds whole, black or white or 1 cup ground chia seeds
- 3 tablespoons unsweetened cocoa powder
- 2 cups unsweetened Almond Breeze Almond Milk (or original if not keto)
- 2 tablespoons Natural Peanut butter
- 1/4 cup Sugar-free flavored maple syrup or any liquid sweetener you like (maple syrup, agave, brown rice syrup) 1/2 teaspoon Vanilla essence
- 1/4 teaspoon Salt

## Instructions

1. Place the chia seed into a blender and blend for about 20 seconds to form ground chia seeds.

2. Add all the rest of the ingredients - order doesn't matter.

3. Blend again for 30 seconds to 1 minute until all the ingredients come together. If it sticks to the sides of the blender, you can stop the blender every 30 seconds, scrape down the side, and repeat until smooth. You can't over-process it!

4. Taste and adjust texture and sweetness. Add more almond milk, 1 tablespoon at a time for a runnier pudding. This may be useful if you replace the sugar-free liquid sweetener with crystal sweetener (erythritol or monk fruit sugar).

5. Transfer into ramekin or serving jar. Decorate with a dollop of fresh peanut butter, drizzle melted sugar-free dark chocolate and chopped peanuts.

6. Enjoy immediately or refrigerate for at least 1 hour for a fresher pudding.

7. Store for up to 4 days in the fridge in an airtight container.

## Nutrition Info

Calories 203 Calories from Fat 111 Fat 12.3g19%

Carbohydrates 24.5g Fiber 19.6g82% Sugar 0.7g1% Protein 6.4g

# Milkshake ice pops

**Prep:**10 mins plus 4 hrs freezing, no cook easy Makes 4

## Ingredients

- 405ml can light condensed milk
- 1 tsp vanilla bean paste
- 1 ripe chopped banana
- 10 strawberries or 3 tbsp  chocolate hazelnut spread

## Directions:

1. Pour the light condensed milk into a food processor and add the vanilla bean paste and chopped banana. Whizz until smooth. Add either the strawberries or chocolate hazelnut spread and whizz again.
2. Divide the mixture between 4 paper cups, cover with foil, then push a lolly stick through the foil lid of each cup until you hit the base. Freeze for 4 hrs or until solid. Will keep in the freezer for 2 months.

# Whisky & pink peppercorn marmalade kit Easy

## Ingredients

- 500g mix of oranges, clementines and lemons
- 1kg demerara sugar
- small pot of pink peppercorns
- small bottle of whisky
- Optional extras
- jam pan muslin
- large wooden spoon
- small jars and labels (makes about 1kg jam)
- To use kit see tip

## Directions:

1. To use the kit:
2. Write the following instructions on the gift tag:Halve the fruits and squeeze the juices into a large saucepan. Remove all the peel and set aside. Put the flesh in the pan with 1 litre water and boil for 15 mins. Push through a sieve lined with muslin and return the liquid to the pan.

3. Shred the peel and tip into a heatproof bowl. Add enough water to just cover and microwave for 3-4 mins until soft. Add the peel to the pan, then add the sugar. Boil for 35-45 mins until the marmalade has reached setting point (keep an eye on it so it doesn't bubble over).

4. Remove from the heat and add 1 tsp pink peppercorns. Allow the mixture to cool a little, then stir in 50ml whisky. Ladle into sterilised jars and seal. Will keep for up to one year.

# *Simnel muffins*

**Prep:**45 mins - 55 mins easy Makes 12

## Ingredients

- 250g mixed dried fruit
- grated zest and juice 1 medium orange
- 175g softened butter
- 175g golden caster sugar
- 3 eggs , beaten
- 300g self-raising flour
- 1 tsp mixed spice
- ½ tsp freshly grated nutmeg
- 5 tbsp milk
- 175g marzipan
- 200g icing sugar
- 2 tbsp orange juice for mixing
- mini eggs

**Directions:**

1. Tip the fruit into a bowl, add the zest and juice and microwave on medium for 2 minutes (or leave to soak for 1 hour). Line 12 deep muffin tins with paper muffin cases.

2. Preheat the oven to fan 180C/ 160C/gas

3. Beat the butter, sugar, eggs, flour, spices and milk until light and fluffy (about 3-5 minutes) – use a wooden spoon or hand held mixer. Stir the fruit in well. Half fill the muffin cases with the mixture. Divide the marzipan into 12 equal pieces, roll into balls, then flatten with your thumb to the size of the muffin cases. Put one into each muffin case and spoon the rest of the mixture over it. Bake for 25-30 minutes, until risen, golden and firm to the touch. Leave to cool.

4. Beat together the icing sugar and orange juice to make icing thick enough to coat the back of a wooden spoon. Drizzle over the muffins and top with a cluster of eggs. Leave to set. Best eaten within a day of making.

# *Prunes Cake*

**Prep time**:20 min Cooking Time: 50min serve: 2

## Ingredients

- ¼ cup vegetable oil
- ¼ cup honey
- 1 egg
- 2 cups coconut flour
- ½ teaspoon salt
- 1 teaspoon baking powder
- 1 cup coconut milk
- 1 teaspoon vanilla extract
- ¼ teaspoon almond extract
- 2 cups chopped prunes, divided
- ¼ cup water
- 1 tablespoon lemon juice

## Instructions

1. Spray two 8-inch round cake pans with vegetable oil spray.

2. In a medium bowl, sift together coconut flour, salt and baking powder. Set aside.

3. In a large mixing bowl, making cream add vegetable oil with the honey until fluffy. Add egg and beat well. Add flour mixture coconut milk. Fold in vanilla and almond extracts and 1 cup chopped prunes.

4. Pour water into Pressure Pot. Place wire trivet into the bottom of the pot and set the pan on top. Place lid on pot and lock into place to seal. Pressure Cook or Manual on High Pressure for 30 minutes. Let sit 10 minutes. Use Quick Pressure Release. Keep cake aside.

5. To make the filling: In an Pressure pot, combine reaming chopped prunes, honey, and water and lemon juice. Close the lid of Pressure pot, Pressure Cook or Manual on High Pressure for 20 minutes. Let sit 10 minutes. Use Quick Pressure Release. Spread thinly between cooled cake layers and on top.

**Nutrition Facts**

Calories 316, Total Fat 23.9g, Saturated Fat 12.7g, Cholesterol 33mg, Sodium 256mg, Total Carbohydrate 77.2g, Dietary Fiber 4.9g, Total Sugars 28.9g, Protein 8.2g

# *Butternut squash Almond Cookies*

**Prep time**: 40 min Cooking Time: 25 min serve: 2

## Ingredients

- 1 cup butter, soften
- ¼ cup honey
- 1 egg, beaten
- ¼ teaspoon vanilla extract
- 1 cup butternut squash. puree
- 2 cups coconut flour
- 1 teaspoon baking powder
- 1 teaspoon baking soda
- ¼ teaspoon salt
- 1 teaspoon ground nutmeg
- ¼ cup walnuts

## Instructions

1. Line the Pressure Pot with parchment paper and spray with nonstick coconut oil spray. Set aside.

2.  Cream together the butter and honey.

3.  Beat together the egg, vanilla and butternut squash puree.

4.  Sift together the coconut flour, baking powder, baking soda, salt and nutmeg; combine with butternut squash mixture and stir in almond.

5.  Add the cookie dough to the prepared Pressure pot. Using a rubber spatula, spread and press the dough into the bottom of the pot, making sure to cover the bottom completely and filling in any gaps.

6.  Cover and lock the lid, but leave the steam release handle in the Venting position. Select High pressure and set the cook time for 15 min. When the cook time is complete, press Cancel to turn off the pot.

7.  Open the lid and carefully transfer the inner pot with the cookie to a cooling rack. Allow the cookie to cool in the pot for a minimum of 30 minutes or until it reaches room temperature.

## Nutrition Facts

Calories 193, Total Fat 17.4g, Saturated Fat 10g, Cholesterol 54mg, Sodium 270mg, Total Carbohydrate 8.1g, Dietary Fiber 0.8g , Total Sugars 6.6g, Protein 1.5g

# *Blackberries Compote*

**Prep time**: 15 min

**Cooking Time:** 20 min

 **serve**: 2

## Ingredients

- 4 cups fresh blackberries
- ¼ cup maple syrup
- 1 teaspoon freshly squeezed lemon juice
- 1 teaspoon orange juice

## Instructions

1. Wash all the blackberries.
2. Add the blackberries and maple syrup to the Pressure Pot. Add the lemon juice and orange juice
3. Lock the lid in place. Select Pressure Cook or Manual, and adjust the pressure to High and the time to 2 minutes. After cooking, let the pressure release naturally for 10 minutes, then quickly release any remaining pressure.

4. Unlock the lid. Taste the berries (carefully—they're hot) and adjust the sweetness if necessary.

**Nutrition Facts**

Calories 250, Total Fat 1.5g, Saturated Fat 0.1g, Cholesterol 0mg, Sodium 7mg, Total Carbohydrate

54.4g, Dietary Fiber 15.3g , Total Sugars 37.5g, Protein 4g

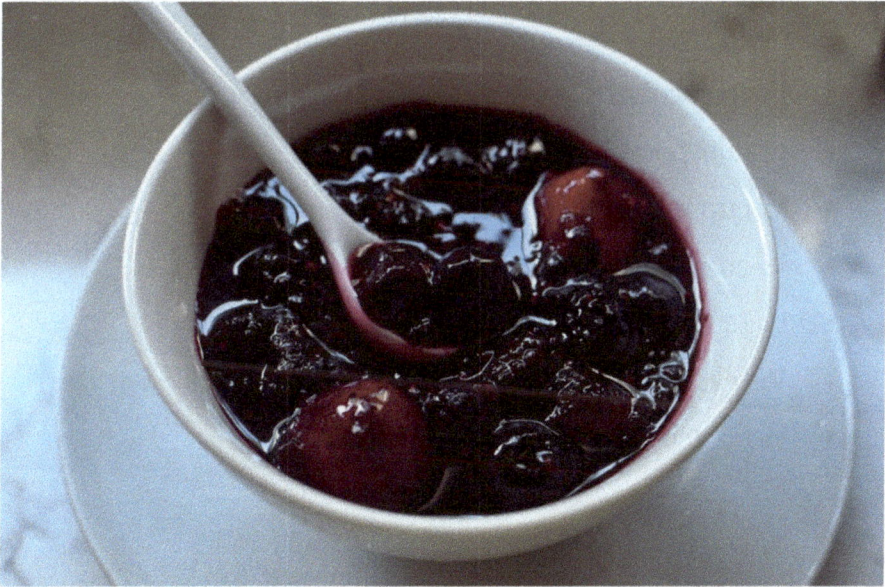

# Raspberry-Vanilla Barley Pudding

**Prep time**: 10 min

**Cooking Time**: 45 min

**serve**: 2

## Ingredients

- 1 cup water
- 1 cup coconut milk
- 1 tablespoon honey
- ½ cup raspberries fresh
- ½ cup barley
- ¼ teaspoon nutmeg
- ¼ teaspoon vanilla
- ½ cup coconut cream

## Instructions

1. Select Sauté on the Pressure Pot and adjust to normal. Add the coconut milk, water, honey, to the pot.

2. Press cancel. Stir in the barley and nutmeg and vanilla into the pot. Secure the lid on the Pressure Pot.

3. Close the pressure-release valve. Select porridge. When cooking is complete, use a natural-release to depressurize.

Remove and Stir in fresh raspberries and cream.

## Nutrition Facts

Calories 502,Total Fat 29.9g, Saturated Fat 25.7g, Cholesterol 0mg , Sodium 28mg, Total Carbohydrate

49.3g, Dietary Fiber 10.7g, Total Sugars 13.2g, Protein 8.5g

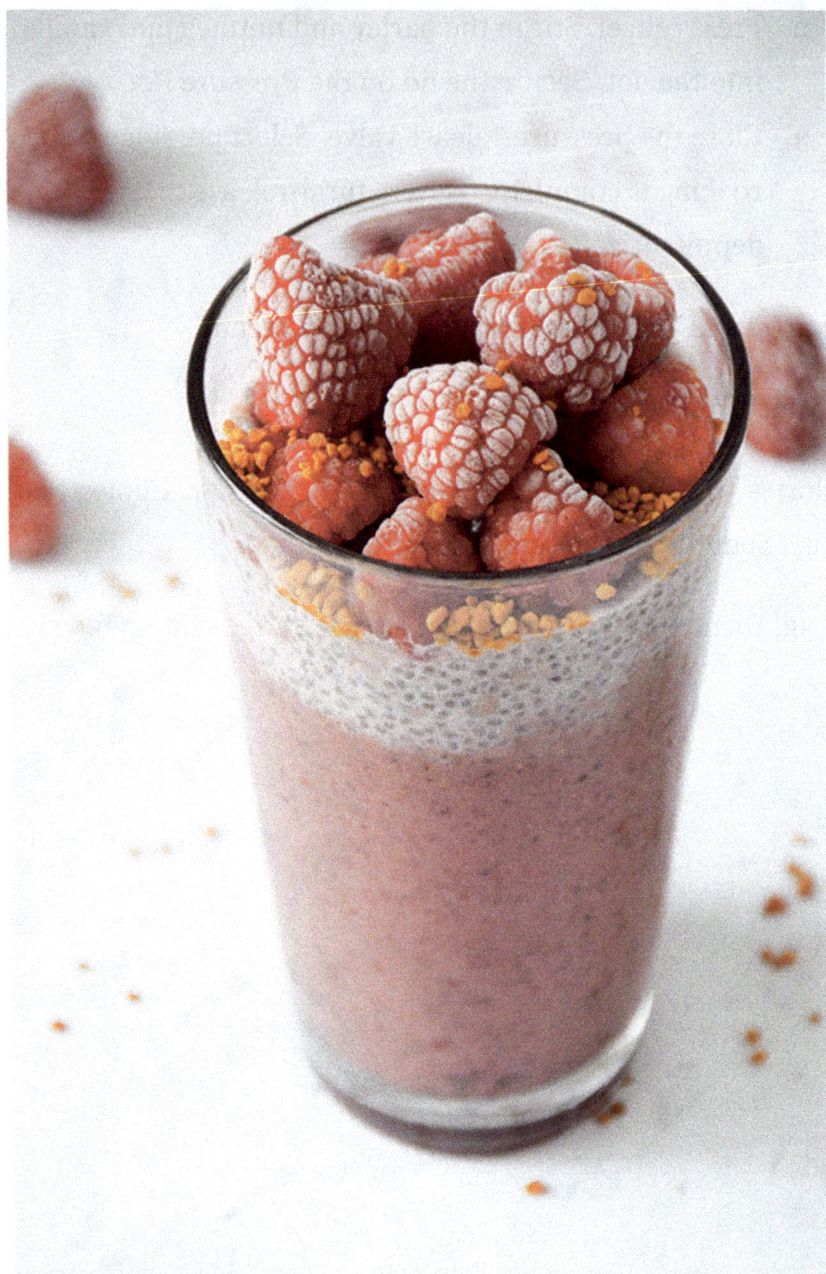